Robbers of the Mind

Robbers of the Mind

JOAN WRENN

authorHOUSE®

AuthorHouse™
1663 Liberty Drive
Bloomington, IN 47403
www.authorhouse.com
Phone: 1-800-839-8640

© 2012 by Joan Wrenn. All rights reserved.

No part of this book may be reproduced, stored in a retrieval system, or transmitted by any means without the written permission of the author.

Published by AuthorHouse   03/17/2012

ISBN: 978-1-4685-6022-0 (sc)
ISBN: 978-1-4685-6023-7 (e)

Library of Congress Control Number: 2012904358

Any people depicted in stock imagery provided by Thinkstock are models, and such images are being used for illustrative purposes only.
Certain stock imagery © Thinkstock.

This book is printed on acid-free paper.

Because of the dynamic nature of the Internet, any web addresses or links contained in this book may have changed since publication and may no longer be valid. The views expressed in this work are solely those of the author and do not necessarily reflect the views of the publisher, and the publisher hereby disclaims any responsibility for them.

ACKNOWLEDGMENTS

I want to thank everyone who encouraged me to write this book. Dr. Sarah Ringel was one of the first who suggested that I put on paper what I had learned about Dementia. Other doctors, social workers, nurses, local Hospice staff, and my family wanted me to write the book so that others who are touched by this dreaded disease would have a compassionate guide while on their journey. I pray that those who read this book will learn from my experience, and from the stories of real people and their struggles.

I am grateful to Jan Slagell for her invaluable editing and friendship. Also, I want to thank my husband for his patience, and my brother, Dace, who was so strong in our sadness.

Joan Wrenn

TABLE OF CONTENTS

Part I
An Introduction to Dementia

Robbers Of The Mind 1

Senile 4

Reality 7

A Day In The Life Of Sharon 12

Health Aliments Typical In The Elderly 17

Part II
Taking Action

As Your Parent Ages, Expect
    And Prepare For Failing Health 25

Use All Available Resources 30

Adjusting To Living In A
    Campus-Like Atmosphere 34

Take Action 39

Anne And Carl 42

Robert's Family Asked, "Why?" 47

Keeping Mother In Her Own Home 52

Time Out For Caregivers 56

Have You Been Diagnosed? 61

The Deep Well Of Forgetfulness 64
Depending On Sitters To Care For Your Parent..... 69

Part III
Day to Day Care

Dementia Cannot Be Delayed Or Cured.................... 75
The Doctor And Pharmacist
    Are Friends You Need 80
Caring For Your Parent At Home 84
Frank Lost Himself 87
When The System Breaks Down................................... 92
Brenda's Last Days 94
Help When You Need It... 99
Glossary Of Words
    Pretaining To Elderly Patient.............................. 102

Blessed in Aging

Blessed are they who understand
My faltering step and shaking hand
Blessed, who know my ears today
Must strain to hear the things they say.

Blessed are those who seem to know
My eyes are dim and my mind is slow.
Blessed are those who look away
When I spilled tea that weary day.

Blessed are they who, with cheery smile
Stopped to chat for a little while
Blessed are they who know the way
To bring back memories of yesterday.

Blessed are those who never say
"You've told that story twice today."
Blessed are they who make it known
That I am loved, respected and not alone.

And blessed are they who will ease the days
Of my journey home, in loving ways.
By Esther Mary Walker

FOREWARD

Writing about people you know and love can be *a piece of cake.* There are fun times and great memories to celebrate with words. Happy times bring memories to embrace for years and years. Memories woven into tall-tales have passed through the centuries since the beginning of civilization.

We find that we would rather not speak of illnesses and the deaths of our family members and friends. Sad memories are difficult to discuss.

It is my hope that as you read this book, you will see that trying to understand the disease of Dementia is very frustrating. No two people follow a downward spiral the same, nor do they fall into perfect steps or stages of the disease as people have listed them. As you will see, each patient is different, and no two days are alike. Being a caregiver to someone close to you who has Dementia is heartbreaking. You ask the doctors all the right questions, but you don't want to believe their answers. Yet every few days, you see a change in your loved one. It may be a subtle sign at first, then many others that break through your denial.

My brother and I traveled down the same road as so many have. We did all we could do to care for Mother, with the help of hired caregivers and Hospice. We did our best to show her our love and support. We were rewarded by her smiles and kisses. We knew that we had done all that could be done, one day at a time.

PREFACE

I have always enjoyed being with older people. When I was three years old, my baby sitter was a lady who lived across the street. She had grey hair, and she always wore an apron over her housedress. Early each morning she came to care for me while Mother and Dad went to work. When I awoke she dressed me for the day and made breakfast for me. Then we crossed one of the busiest streets in town to reach her house. Our routine of the day began as we climbed the steep steps to her large front porch. Mrs. Clapp lifted me into a big white swing and sat down beside me. She talked about the traffic, and spoke to the ladies as they passed by. She read to me and sang songs. Her voice was sweet to my ears even though I noticed slight tremors and crackles as she spoke.

After lunch, Mrs. Clapp and I walked down the sidewalk to visit some of the neighbors. There was one old man always dressed in black who lived three houses down. Even I saw the hump on his back as he bent over the machine knitting socks. White socks were everywhere. Farther down the street, we usually visited an older lady who was very ill. Mrs. Clapp always took something good to eat for the families' supper. We visited until the three teenage children came home from school.

Two years later my parents moved to a more rural neighborhood. An older lady with white hair visited with us often, and my dad's parents lived close by. While mother worked, my grandparents took care of me. Granny took me to the garden with her where I helped pick up potatoes while she gathered squash, tomatoes, and beans for dinner. I went with granddaddy to feed the pigs and watched him milk the cows. Granny and I were very close, probably because I was constantly at her heels. She talked to me about her flowers, and worked in them often. Granddaddy thought that time was wasted working in flowers. He often said, "You should be working to raise food to feed the large family we have."

Granny would answer, "These flowers are food for the soul and don't you forget it."

As time passed, Mother quit her job and stayed at home with me. We visited my grandparents several times a week, and Granny even spent some time at our house when my baby brother was born. She never lost her love for flowers. She planted a dogwood tree and some buttercups around our house. Her plants never needed to be replanted. Her pretty flowers fed all our souls.

This gentle lady lived to see her seven children grown and married. She baby sat several grandchildren and raised three others. But as she grew older, granny changed. She had problems recognizing her children and grandchildren. She repeated words over and over. Wherever she was she wanted to "go home". She could not bathe or care for herself.

One day, dear Granny took to her bed and closed her eyes. Her family gathered and whispered among themselves. The doctor arrived, took her pulse and listened to her heart. The grown-ups met with the doctor in the kitchen and returned wiping tears. I held her hand and sang to her until she could hear me no more.

Part I

An Introduction to Dementia

ROBBERS OF THE MIND

Many years ago there was a lady living in our neighborhood who started acting strange and out of character. I had known her and her family most of my life. We attended church together. At first, it was hard to decide what made her so different. I could not understand why I was so uncomfortable when in her company. I later heard that she was "forgetful."

This lady drove around aimlessly for many months with no real destination in mind. Sometimes she would stop by my mother's house for a visit. She, very casually, would stroll up the steps, open the door and walk in. She greeted no one by name, but proceeded to sit on the sofa and talk about her family and all the things they were doing. Any comment we made was ignored as she talked nonstop. When she looked at us, we could see no recognition in her eyes. After fifteen or twenty minutes, she would stand up, walk to the door and leave without another word.

This was my first encounter with Dementia, but I didn't know it at the time. The lady's family realized what a danger she was to herself and others. They took her to several doctors. Each doctor talked about how poor their mother's cognitive skills were. They all suggested that the mother should be admitted to a local nursing home. Her children found a facility that would take elderly people with emotional and mental problems. The staff called the condition senility or hardening of the arteries. The nurses did all they could do to give the mother the of best care. However, they were perplexed by her violence, bad language, and her tendency to tear off her clothes at any point in time.

In the past two or three decades, people have become more aware of Dementia. We know that there are many kinds of Dementia, and we all know someone who is affected by it. The good news is that nursing homes are more prepared to deal with patients with

Dementia. Many times half the facility is dedicated to the care of our loved ones who have symptoms of this disease. In addition, there are web sites devoted to helping families find suitable care for their relatives.

Some good sites are:

www.aplaceformom.com
www.familycaregiversonline.com

SENILE

Forget the word *senile*. Senile is a word used frequently in years passed to describe the forgetfulness and strange behavior of our grandparents. The correct word in use now is *Dementia*. Dementia generally means a breakdown of communication within the brain. Simply stated: Signals are crossed and going to all the wrong places. As a patient begins to make a comment, unrelated thoughts intrude leading to words that make no sense and are far away from their intended response.

The brain is a wonderfully made and finely tuned organ, but as we age our brain changes. It shrinks in size and weight causing forgetfulness and a decrease in our cognitive function. Cognition means to "know." In the natural process of aging, our cognitive abilities diminish to a certain extent. We know things because of the skills of perception, reasoning, attention, judgment, memory and intuition. When something goes wrong with the wiring that triggers these, the brain cannot respond to the hundreds of messages it receives.

When there is a disorder or severe impairment of the brain, you may lose your independence and the ability to care for your personal needs. Dementia has many faces. Alzheimer's is the most well-known; followed by Vascular Dementia, Parkinson's disease and Huntington's disease.

Dementia is the decline of the mental functions of the brain. Since no one knows the cause and there is no cure, living with Dementia presents a challenge for the patient, his family and his caregivers. Learning to live each day as it comes and having a strong faith is the only therapy for this disease. There is, thankfully, medicine to calm anxieties and help patients sleep at night.

When an early diagnosis is made there is enough time to plan and discuss what lies ahead for everyone involved. Accept the fact that no two days will be alike. Also know that you are helpless. There is nothing to be done except calm the fears, stress and frustration of a patient suffering from one of the many faces of Dementia.

REALITY

I opened my eyes, stretched and wondered what the weatherman had predicted for today. I don't remember watching the news last night. Why? Then reality took over. I know why I missed the news. I was with mom late into the night while we were getting her settled at the hospital. Dan, my brother, stayed the remainder of the night, and I drove home—worried and tired. My thoughts were: "This is my world now—a world of doctors, nurses, pills, hospitals, nursing homes, late nights, and many, many prayers". I threw back the cover, hurriedly, slipped on my shoes and went to the kitchen to make coffee. Charles had let me sleep while he worked outside before the heat of summer set in. I heard the mower in the distance (far away from the house so as not to wake me), and I started a quick breakfast of toast, eggs and bacon.

I knew that I needed to shower and rush to the hospital. My dear mother had endured yet another fall, even while my daughter was in the same room with her. Try as we may, none of us could get her to use her walker. This was her third fall in six months to require emergency treatment. Later, as the warm water refreshed my body, I asked for strength and energy to help care for my ninety-one year old mother.

Mother began falling, over a year ago, causing little bruises and achy muscles. She was taken to ER for stitches to her head and an evaluation. The next time she fell was when she tried to enter her home, but fell backward instead. This last fall caused a broken hip, and the operation was to be today. Even though all the doctors cautioned her to use a cane or walker, Mom refused.

We tried physical therapy to improve her balance, and we consulted geriatric physicians, as well as her primary care physician. All of them told her she must use a walking aid. But to no avail. Her refusal to use help while walking may have been part of an underlying problem that was surfacing gradually.

Two years prior to this last fall, Mother had become more and more afraid of being alone at night. She would not admit any fear and refused to move in with Charles and me. She always said: "Joyce, you and I are too much alike, and we would never get along. Besides, there's no place like home." I knew that she was right, but when she began calling me at night about strange noises, people in her house and a small child being lost in her house, I knew we needed a plan.

My brother and I agreed to alternate nights sleeping at mom's house so that we all could get some sleep. She did seem to sleep better, but she still saw things that we could not see, and she continued to hear voices. We reassured Mom that one of us was in the guest room nearby, and she could call out if she needed anything. We continued sleeping over for about two years.

Mother followed her old routine of rising at 6am and fixing breakfast for my brother, Dan and herself. He had to be at work by 8am, and Mother thought that he never ate right unless she saw him eat his favorites that she lovingly prepared. As the years passed, this task took longer each morning. However, it gave her a reason to get up and do something worthwhile. Our father was gone, and we were glad for her determination.

The biggest problem was getting her to use her walking aids. Even though she was not steady on her feet, as soon as she reached the kitchen, the cane found a corner.

It was in the kitchen where she fell and broke her hip. The doctor who operated on her hip expected Mom's health to decline rapidly, and suggested the constant care of a nursing home. A few days later an ambulance transported mom to a large facility where she could receive therapy. She was placed in a double room, but she could not understand why her roommate was always talking. The lady tried to be nice to mom, but nothing would do but to move her to a private room.

The routine was so fast paced and busy in the nursing home. Quick baths, rushed visits to the toilet, and someone was always waiting to take her to physical therapy, the dining room or a scheduled activity. It took us all a while to get used to the fast pace. Sometimes, mother would refuse to leave her room for therapy or other activities. Everything was so new and confusing; she wanted someone to stay with her at all times. We were there in the morning; we helped take her to lunch and paid a sitter to spend the afternoon. We returned at night to be sure she was in bed and asleep. All the changes pushed mother farther into the Dementia that had been increasing each year. Thankfully, the doctors had prepared us for this also.

A DAY IN THE LIFE OF SHARON

It's early in the morning and Sharon is getting out her clothes for church services. She had been thinking since early morning about what to wear. Her clothes were color coordinated so that she could select easily, but she could not make a decision. The more she looked in the closet, the more confused she got. Sharon wondered where all her favorite clothes were. Finally, she called her daughter (for the third time since 6am), and asked her what to wear to church today. And for the third time, Jenny told her that today is not Sunday. Tomorrow is Sunday.

Sharon pretended to remember their earlier conversations. She then began to accuse Jenny of taking her clothes and wearing them. After all, Jenny had been moving clothes around in her closet one day. She continued to berate her daughter or tell Jenny how ungrateful she was. How thoughtless she was. She told Jenny that she didn't care about anyone but herself. Sharon asked Jenny why she never visited.

Jenny quietly wiped away tears as her mother continued to scold her and whip her with words. She tried to interrupt Sharon and explain that she had never taken her clothes. She had only tried to help by putting her closet in order for easy selection. Jenny reminded her mother that she would stop by this afternoon and help her decide on an outfit for church tomorrow. In the background, Jenny heard her mom's smoke alarm screaming. Jenny called a neighbor of her mother's for help, and ran to her car.

When Jenny pulled into the driveway of the small brick house that was home for twenty years, she found her mother in a rocking chair on the back porch. Sharon seemed calm and unaffected. Jenny rushed into the kitchen and found the neighbor turning on fans and opening windows. The house was full of smoke because a frying pan of bacon caught on fire. When the neighbor arrived, Sharon was taking the blazing pan outside. Jenny began cleaning up the residue of smoke on the stove and cabinets. Her hands were trembling just thinking of the close call that was barely avoided. The neighbor left after Jenny told her how thankful she was for her help. Then Jenny turned to see her mother biding her neighbor good-bye as though nothing had happened.

Jenny moved to the familiar back porch. This was the porch where her mother and father had enjoyed the evening sunsets together. The rocking chairs were perfect for lingering with a date before that goodnight kiss. Good memories flooded her mind. Her eyes met Sharon's eyes. For a minute, Jenny saw something different. Did her mother know her? She was so quiet and reserved. She told herself that her Mom was still shaken because there was almost a serious fire. Well, at least, she was not angry anymore. Jenny sat down beside her mother and took her hand. Sharon looked confused. She asked Jenny why was she there. Jenny started to explain what had happened. Her mother looked puzzled. They sat there a long time, rocking and holding hands. Jenny took a deep breath, and let it out quietly. She knew that she must call her sisters and then the doctor.

So many times it's scenes like the previous one that brings us to an "ah-ha" moment. We know that there is something wrong, but what? She began by losing things and spending all day rambling through drawers. Sharon was fearful of being alone at night. She heard voices, saw people who were not there and looked for a baby that was lost. Sharon knew that she was in trouble, but she didn't want her family to know. She learned how to change a subject if she was lost for words, and she covered well when she could not call a friend by name. Sharon took it well when she was told she could not drive anymore, however, she refused to sign a power of attorney paper, and was very suspicious when her children tried to help her with business matters.

Dementia gives no warning. It's nothing we expect, and reality hits us between the eyes when a diagnosis is made. Dementia is an illness that robs the mind of wonderful memories, and leaves a shell of a person who is fearful, agitated, paranoid, verbally (and sometimes physically) abusive, forgetful and who cannot carry on a conversation. But the Dementia patient is someone's beloved mother, father, sister or brother and, he or she deserves to feel the love and security that can only be shown by a family member. A family member or members usually take on the role of caregiver when Dementia is declared the culprit that is slowly stealing a loved one's mind. It is a sad and demanding roll. Being a Caregiver is a big challenge that requires research, and hands-on attention.

The Primary Care Physician is the first step on the ladder of learning about Dementia. Hopefully, this doctor has previous healthcare knowledge of your loved one. He should be able to give informal tests to the patient, and conduct an interview that should shed light on her mental state. Family members need to speak privately with the doctor about their loved one's behavior. They should listen carefully to the doctor's comments and suggestions and take notes. The PCP may refer the patient to a geriatric physician who specializes in aliments of the elderly.

HEALTH ALIMENTS TYPICAL IN THE ELDERLY

A large part of our population is now considered elderly. Due to the many advances of modern medicine, people are living well into their nineties. But the bad news is that most of these elders are suffering from illnesses that cause them to be home-bound or confined to nursing homes. The most common ailments affecting our maturing population are:

- Dementia (Alzheimer's, and/or strokes caused by narrowed arteries)
- Heart problems (CAD, heart failure, vascular problems including blood clots)
- COPD (Chronic Obstructive Pulmonary Disease)
- Cancers of all kinds
- Mental Illness (depression, brain damage) classically due to loneliness, loss of independence, multiple health

problems and side effects of medications used to treat them.
- Falls resulting in broken hips, broken legs, etc. usually begin a down-hill process in health.

I don't pretend to be a health professional, but these health problems are the ones I have observed in my family and friends. Furthermore, I won't use clinical terms. Since knowledge is power and understanding enables us to use that power, I pray that readers will find comfort and strength as they struggle to be good caretakers to their loved ones. There is a glossary at the back to help us all converse more intelligently with health professionals.

In reference to the illnesses mentioned above, Dementia is the one with which I am most familiar. I have consulted doctors, the Internet, other caretakers, nurses, therapist and read many articles, but nothing replaces knowing how to cope day—to day and knowing what to expect. Some of the behaviors described can apply to many aliments that affect the elderly.

Also, there are several kinds of Dementia, and I will write about them as a layman.

Dealing with Dementia is heart breaking and differs with each person. A mild, soft-spoken person may change by 180 degrees, or show mild to moderate personality changes. Many of these changes are caused as your loved one fights feelings of helplessness and frustration. As the ability to carry on a meaningful conversation begins to fade, your loved one knows something is terribly wrong. A more demanding, controlling parent may become meek and very cooperative. He may wonder aloud why he cannot remember something. He may use unrelated words in a sentence, and wonder why no one understands him. He may realize that the words are wrong and try to cover up by laughing or crying. Your loved one may eventually stop trying and remain silent. Depression often takes over.

We, as potential caretakers, must be aware of early signs that we see as unusual. The signs are subtle, but we must take them seriously.

Pay attention to when a parent begins to do the following:

1. Loose things more than you do.
2. Forget the names of friends and some family members.
3. See things that are not there, for instance: children swinging from a chandelier, strangers standing around her bed, hearing voices like a radio is playing, and looking for lost babies.
4. Be afraid to be at home alone at night.
5. Forget, temporarily, where she is.
6. Shows other signs of paranoia and/or hallucinations.
7. Loose interest in hobbies and social activities.
8. Displays mood and personality changes.
9. Loses track of time.
10. Forgets recently acquired information.

Parents need comfort and love during this frightening time. We found it helpful to have a family member spend each night on a rotating basis. We could hear mother when she got up at night and see that she returned to her bed safely. Mother had experienced falls recently, so it was even more important to watch her at night. She became calmer, less anxious, and more like her old self within a few days. She also began sleeping much better. This was the beginning of mom's Dementia.

Part II
Taking Action

AS YOUR PARENT AGES, EXPECT AND PREPARE FOR FAILING HEALTH

We soon realized that Mom needed more than comfort and a peaceful night's rest. She lost a very expensive hearing aid; she thought people were watching her, and her falls became more frequent and the consequences more serious. Her doctor suggested physical therapy to improve her strength and gait. The PT encouraged her to use her cane or her walker.

My brother and I continued to stay with her at night, help her make breakfast, make her bed, and sweep and vacuum the floors. I checked in on her three or four times a day because I live next door. I took her grocery shopping while she supported herself by holding the grocery cart. It became an increasingly long and tedious outing because Mom read all the labels, and it took her so long to finally decide what to purchase. I would help her make the final selections and then write her check for her. She always said that her handwriting was so bad, but I think she could not remember how to write the check herself.

She continued to walk without her cane. In addition, she began to fall . . . at first without injury, but then bumps and bruises appeared. We began to realize that falling was a real problem. One day when she was alone, she fell and cut her head on the TV. My nephew found her shortly after she fell. My brother called 911, and she was taken to the hospital where she had several stitches.

We began staying with her for longer periods, and we put her cane beside her chair to remind her to use it. In retrospect, the cane probably would not have helped.

Mom finally told us that she became dizzy and did not remember falling. She fell another time in her home, thankfully with no injuries.

However, with the onset of summer, she could not resist walking a few yards to the garden to pick tomatoes. On this particular day the temperature was 98 degrees in the shade. She lay in the sun for at least 20 minutes while we thought she was taking her usual afternoon nap. When I found her sitting near the door to the porch, I picked her up, and took her into her bedroom. I turned on the fan, turned up the air conditioner and put wet cloths on her face. She could have easily had a heat stroke. Even with all the warning signs I refused to face the facts: Mom needed someone with her 24 hours a day.

Mom's health problems had slowly become worse. So slowly in fact, that we, like other adult children, were able to fool ourselves into believing that everything was okay. Seeing your once-so-active parent become weak and dependent is difficult to witness. We, as potential caretakers, must prepare ourselves and watch for clues that our parents may need help as they grow older and less firm. The truth of the matter is that we should always be observant and meet each challenge as it comes. It is only natural as we grow older, to call someone by the wrong name and fall into periods of depression. It's frustrating to be unable to drive anymore, not to be able to see or hear as well, and most of all, not to be active anymore. Add to that the loss of a spouse or child, then loneliness and loss of joy prevails. The above-mentioned behavior is to be expected as life unfolds around us.

The real signs of health problems are much more severe and should be addressed promptly. As part of being observant of your parent's behavior and health, he/she will have to have regular check-ups with the Primary Care Physician. I believe this is taken for granted. You should make good use of these check-ups by attending the visits with your parent. Any questions you may have about your parent's mental or physical health should be written in a notebook. You should ask the questions, and record the answers. Don't forget to inquire about current medicines, or new meds prescribed. Record your parent's pulse, blood pressure, temperature and weight. At the next appointment, you may notice a difference in some of the readings. Bring this to the doctor's attention. I know there are notes in your parent's charts, but sometimes doctors are so rushed, they don't read everything.

It's been said that a doctor spends less than nine minutes with each patient. Since we have so many patients and so few doctors, this strikes me as a plausible thought. Be very vocal about your parent's health, and be sure you get an answer. If the doctor is unsure about a certain physical ailment affecting your parent, ask for a specialist. The PCP can arrange an appointment for your parent. An aging person with several health issues would also benefit from a Patient Geriatric Evaluation.

USE ALL AVAILABLE RESOURCES

Three years before my mother began to fall, we called Duke Medical Center and requested an appointment with a well-known geriatrician, D., Kenneth Schmader. A Geriatric Evaluation is very thorough, and covers all the bases. A team of doctors and specialists began gathering information from many sources. They heard her complaints, checked all her lab tests, x-rays and CT scans. They looked at her meds, her eyes, her ears, her teeth, listened to her chest, and saw pictures of her heart with stints in place. They gave her a neurological exam, and viewed every inch of her body (stomach, feet, head, back, etc.). They took her temperature, blood pressure, weight and reviewed Mom's diabetic condition.

The doctors said there was mild cognitive impairment, chronic UTIs, unsteady gait, and weight loss as a summary of her problems. They suggested that with regular visits of her family and the use of Lifeline, Mom could continue to live independently. This evaluation was done two years before mom began to fall. Many older men and women seem to easily lose their balance as time goes by. We have an emergency scanner at home, and over half of the calls for emergency medical services usually involve a fall. These falls occur in nursing homes, assisted living facilities, and in private homes.

Most falls involve women rather than men. Most likely because women live longer, and they tend to develop osteoporosis (thinning of the bones). Doctors have expressed to me that a fall involving a broken hip or a broken leg, begins major failing health for the elderly. There will be surgery to repair the damage, an order for physical therapy, and placement in a high level of care nursing home. Being in pain, hospitalized and subjected to physical therapy while adjusting to a different environment can traumatize anyone.

Some of these older men and women become lonely, and depressed. Many won't eat. Health begins to deteriorate. However, there are many courses of action that can turn some of the afore-mentioned situations around. The discharge nurse or caseworker will work from the hospital to insure a placement in a suitable nursing/rehabilitation institution (this is true for anyone who cannot stay alone and needs special care).

Just as everyone has a different DNA, each care facility is unique. The family has the responsibility to investigate a prospective facility before a loved one is placed. We did not know at first that there was a web site that rated each institution based on cleanliness, ratio of patients to caregivers, quality of food, quality of health care given and any complaints that may have been filed against the facility. You may obtain these web sites and see open records by contacting your local Department of Social Services (DSS). They will be glad to answer your questions.

The ultimate goal in most cases is to get the parent back on his/her feet and take them home to familiar surroundings. I have heard elderly people in nursing homes beg and cry to go home. I know in many cases that parents can't go home again. Severe health problems can make it impossible.

While serving on an observation board, I visited many small and large healthcare facilities. We talked to the residents, checked the standards of cleanliness, care, food preparation and looked for safety hazards. When we interviewed those in charge, we learned that it was difficult to engage the residents in planned activities. We saw apathy and depression. Very few residents ever had visitors. We reported our findings to the local Ombusman. He reviewed the problems as we saw them, sent out other inspectors and finally took steps that would benefit the patients and assure their health and safety. If you see or suspect abuse or neglect in any healthcare facility, please contact your local Ombudsman or Department of Social Services.

ADJUSTING TO LIVING IN A CAMPUS-LIKE ATMOSPHERE

While your parent may need to live in a nursing home, she does not have to feel alone and forgotten. There are many ways family and friends can help. If the family is large, a schedule may be made for visitation. At least one person a day should sit and talk with the resident. It does not matter if she/he understands or answers. The main purpose is to keep her familiar with her family. If she smiles, you have been successful. Keep a book in her room so that visitors may sign it. I know of a family who encouraged visitors to jot down the date, time and general mood of the patient. It's a wonderful tool to use so the family can see how the parent's day was spent. Also, reviewing the list of visitors with the parent is a great way to communicate and stimulate awareness and memory.

Many families have found it useful to try to vary the hours they spend at the nursing home. It is important to meet all the nurses/CNA's who are the regular caregivers. Observe what your parent eats, and what kind of medicine she gets. You may even ask to see the lists of meds to be sure it compares with what her PCP prescribed. Make friends with the staff and thank them for all they do to care for your parent. They have a difficult job that requires patience and endurance; and they have a love and concern for their patients. Be kind and show your appreciation for all their hard work. I treasure each kind word spoken to my parent. When shown kindness, our loved ones are not as lonely and they adjust to their new home much quicker.

I have observed several acts of love and kindness many times in the nursing home setting. One petite white haired lady seemed not to mind living with other residents. She was gentle, and she carried on conversations with others around her.

Granted, she never spoke as though she understood what others were saying. However, she seemed content. I believe that she lived each day knowing that she would eat at least two meals a day with a member of the family, her devoted nephew. Twice a day he was there eating lunch and dinner with his proud aunt.

Another lady who was confined to her wheelchair, waited patiently for her afternoon visitor. She would roll herself toward the entrance, or wheel outside on a nice day. She would talk with other residents, or she might fall asleep, but when her daughter drove in, her face lit up. They talked; the daughter pushed her around to admire the flowers, and they ate dinner together. This older lady seemed perfectly adjusted to her surroundings.

Another method that helps your loved one adjust to a new setting is to bring beloved pictures from her home. Hang them on the wall so she can see them. Many will ask about the people in the pictures, and your loved one will enjoy talking about them. I know one lady who had a painting of her home in a blanket of snow hanging over her bed. She told many stories about that beautiful painting. It was so very special to her.

If there is enough space in your parent's room, try bringing a few pieces of furniture, maybe a favorite recliner, a desk, a few lamps, and especially her television. I visited one lady who had her family move her complete bedroom suite into her room. What a great idea!

Encourage friends, relatives and church members to send cards to communicate with your parent. Subscribe to the local paper or a favorite magazine. You might ask friends to give you the reading material they are discarding. Most facilities have small libraries, and even computer rooms. On your visits, put your parent in a wheelchair and visit these sources of information, visit other patients or take her to a planned activity. Some facilities are promoting the Wii as great exercise and mind stimulant. Always view the Activity Chart and ask what's going on.

Siblings should always stay in touch, and take an active interest in their parent's condition. It's sad to see a loved one get weaker and know there is nothing we can do to turn back the *hands of time*. Many believe that these very circumstances could serve as a catalyst that will bring the family together for a common cause. You may feel closer to your siblings than ever before. A special bond forms when a family comes together for the love and concern of a parent.

TAKE ACTION

When a family comes together to make plans for the treatment and care of their parent, there are many things to consider. The present health of the loved one, the recommendations of the primary-care doctor, and how much time each sibling will contribute. This is a time to face the facts and take action that will benefit your parent. His/her future health and well-being is at stake.

Is your parent able to stay at home? Can he/she walk with help? Is there a need for bathing, dressing and meal preparation? Can she stay home with a paid caregiver or will the siblings agree to take turns to do what needs to be done? Other than cooking meals, helping with bathing and dressing, keeping the house fall-proof and clean, keeping all doctor's appointments and keeping clothes and bed linens clean, the caretaker must pick up prescribed meds and arrange them in a large medicine box with days and hour marked. To avoid mistakes with his/her care, a notebook/log should be kept concerning change in meds, any health problems that may occur in the day and other information that may be helpful at doctor's appointments or when a nurse comes to check on your parent. We always recorded Mom's blood sugar, time her insulin was given, if she ate well, and her general mood.

I'm well acquainted with a family of seven siblings. When their mother became very dependent but did not want to leave her home, they came up with a great solution. They discussed the best way to give their Mom loving care, so they made a schedule. Each sibling and spouse chose a twenty-four hour day that suited him/her. All seven days were covered, and everyone knew how to plan his/her week. When families are large, and they all agree to make the sacrifice, caretaking is simplified. I'm sure there were problems, and maybe everyone was not happy all the time, but their dedication never wavered.

I just described an ideal situation. However, families are not large these days; giving up a day each week for years is tough; and I can't think of any other family who has been able to come up with such a unique solution.

ANNE AND CARL

Anne is an eighty-two year old lady who looks as normal as your own grandmother. She has two sons who are not well, and a daughter she seldom sees. Anne's other daughter, Sara, died under suspicious circumstances more than a year ago. Anne lives with her husband, Carl, whom she married while he was still in the Navy. Their four children were born while Carl was serving his country, leaving Anne and the children alone for months at a time. The couple now lives comfortably in a rural area.

I observed Carl and Anne in the grocery store one afternoon. Carl held her hand as they walked very slowly up and down the aisles. They stopped to look at produce or canned food, and Anne had to touch each proposed selection. Carl patiently took the items and placed them in his basket or returned them to the shelves. I heard him numerous times urging Anne to "hurry along." They slowly made their way to the checkout counter. Anne was shuffling along after Carl as they left the store.

Since we had known this couple for some time, we visited one day to see if we could be of help. They were both glad to see us. Anne approached me immediately and wanted to talk. I asked where should we sit, but she looked perplexed, so I took her hand and led her to the sofa. She took both my hands in hers and kept telling me what a good person I am. I asked about her health, and she replied in sentences that really said nothing. She wanted desperately to have a conversation, but she could not understand me, and she could not respond correctly. Carl confided that he was at his wits end. He could not leave Anne alone while he mowed the lawn, took out garbage or cooked their meals. Anne is not interested in TV or reading. She continually paces. She goes to bed very early and gets up each morning a 4:00.

Carl has many needs. The adult children don't come to visit, and they don't offer to help. I doubt that they know how much their mother needs care. Carl has always been a man of quiet strength who could handle many things without help. Now he does not know where to turn. His beloved wife has a dreaded disease called Alzheimer's, and Carl needs all the help he can get.

I was able to point out to Carl that there are Adult Day Care Services available in our area, and I suggested some other sources of help. The Veterans Administration can be of financial help since Carl served in the navy during wartime. And I urged him to ask Anne's doctor to get Home Health Care involved. Also Respite Care is available at local nursing homes. Anne could spend a few days away from home, and Carl would be sure that she would get her meals, her medicine and professional care. As primary caretaker, Carl needs some time off. I reminded Carl that Meals-on-Wheels could also be a great help. Until Carl starts getting outside help, church members and neighbors are sitting with Anne to give Carl time to mow the lawn, keep doctor's appointments and run errands. Friends are also bringing in cooked meals, and food that is easily prepared.

Caring for someone with Dementia is a full-time job. Some spouses feel overwhelmed at the intensity of care they must provide. When the time comes that a loved one cannot be cared for at home, the spouse and children often feel like they are betraying their spouse/parent by placing them in a nursing home. Just remember that Dementia is responsible for draining all the strength, patience and good health from many caretakers.

After several months of being the sole caretaker, Carl was beginning to experience chest pains and made numerous visits to his doctor. His condition was one that would require surgery. Carl considered the options. He finally moved Anne to a local nursing home, which provided a Memory Care Unit. Anne is still her pleasant self, and she took the move very well. Now, Carl can take care of his problems.

We have all heard of Alzheimer's disease, and it is but one of the many kinds of

Dementia. Vascular Dementia is second only to Alzheimer's disease, causing the loss of cognitive reasoning and thinking abilities. With Alzheimer's disease, from the first signs of Dementia to the person's death ranges from 7 to 10 years. However, there is no sure diagnosis of Dementia of any kind until the brain can be autopsied after death. Some symptoms are the same for several kinds of Dementia.

Dementia of any type is a cruel disease that robs many of our loved ones of precious memories. Words that could have been spoken are locked forever in minds that once held love and affection for families who are now heartbroken. The reality is that there is no cure. There is nothing we can do but keep our loved ones clean, well fed and free from bodily danger. The vacant look in eyes that used to speak of pride and love makes us know just how helpless we are in the path of this deteriorating disease.

ROBERT'S FAMILY ASKED, "WHY?"

Robert lives with his wife, and they are both retired. He tends a small garden each summer, and delights in giving the fruits of his labor to his son and neighbors. During the past two or three years, Robert's wife has noticed some changes in his personality. She told herself that they were getting older, and forgetfulness is only natural. Except lately, Robert would lose things and blame her. He seemed nervous, and his language was riddled with curse words. She spoke with their son, James, when Robert began locking up the house like a fortress. He even kept a baseball bat in a corner and a hatchet under the bed.

James took his father to the family doctor. Robert resisted and did not cooperate very well when the doctor was asking questions. He was clever with his answers, and accused James and his wife of being crazy. The doctor was able to calm him. He prescribed medication for his agitation, and medicine to slow down his obvious history of Dementia. The doctor explained to James in private about his father's prognosis. Each stage would present new problems, and it seemed that Robert was slipping into the second level of this dreaded mental disorder.

The doctor suggested that his mother needed help coping with Robert's illness. He warned that his behavior would decline, and soon outside care would be needed. As the months and years progress, Robert may walk off and forget how to return home. He will not know his old friends and sometimes not even his family. His anger and agitation could cause him to be a danger to himself and others. Robert may fall and break a bone, he will eventually have to wear diapers, he may tear paper and magazines into strips, he will rub, pat, clap or bang on things for no reason. He will not be able to converse with others because he will not understand, and he won't remember the correct words to use.

James was shocked by what the doctor had said. He wondered where to start. With the new medicine, maybe Robert could adapt to a daycare atmosphere. That would give his Mom a rest for a few hours each week. She could do her shopping without Robert walking behind and complaining. She could also get away to get her hair done as she had for years. Now to break the news to his mother that her life would never be the same again.

James and his mother were able to get an adult daycare to care for Robert three days a week, for a few hours each day. There he was exposed to storytelling, games, painting and music. In the beginning, he really did not want to go, but after he went a few times, it wasn't so bad. They kept his hands and mind busy, but he was still suspicious of everyone. Robert enjoyed the music, and after he got home, he would walk and sing. However, he became disruptive and began taking things that belonged to others. His conversation skills were limited, and he mumbled a lot. After several months, James and his mother decided to keep Robert at home.

While Robert was going to adult care, James set about finding two people trained in nursing skills to help his mother take care of Robert. They helped him bathe, dress and tried to keep him mobile with a walker and a wheelchair. They were needed now more than ever. Each night, after Robert was safely in bed the helper would leave.

Then something unexpected happened. James came by his parents' home as he did early each day. Before the aid arrived, James usually helped his father out of the bed and helped him with other personal things while his mother made breakfast.

But this Friday, James walked in to a nightmare.

He found his mother badly beaten. Robert was walking around aimlessly mumbling and singing. He still carried the bat. James called 911 and went with his mother to the hospital just as the male aid arrived. The aid cleaned up Robert and the bloody mess in the bedroom. He gave Robert his breakfast and his medications.

He helped Robert to his recliner where he fell fast asleep.

James stayed by his mother's side as she was examined. She begged him not to call the police. She told James how his father was so frightened at night. He heard and saw things that were not there. On this particular night, he awoke and thought someone had broken into the house. Robert got out of bed, and began swinging the bat at his wife with amazing strength as she returned from the bathroom. She tried to stop him, but Robert seemed super strong in his fear. Robert was taken to a nursing home that was equipped to handle people in the latter stages of Dementia. His wife slowly recovered but was left wheelchair bound. James and his mother visited Robert in the nursing home every day, even though he could not talk and he did not seem to know them.

What a heart-breaking true story. In all cases of Dementia hearts are breaking every day. Our loved ones are suffering, and there's not much we can do except see that they are well fed, clean, comfortable and loved.

KEEPING MOTHER IN HER OWN HOME

I spoke with a friend of mine as we both rushed out from choir practice.

I wondered why she was in such a hurry. We stopped for a minute to talk, and she told me her experience with Dementia. It sounded a lot like mine.

She was hurrying to her mother's house to help do her part to care for her. This 50's something busy mother had spent the last ten years helping her brother make their mom's life as comfortable and peaceful as possible. When symptoms first appeared and a diagnosis was made, her mom was in her early seventies. A family conference was held to decide alternatives for her health care. The decision was to "keep mother home."

Here was another strong family who was willing to sacrifice their time and energy for the sake of their mom's care. Sure, there was a lot of planning to do, but they were dedicated to keeping her in a peaceful, familiar atmosphere. Two siblings cannot accomplish this difficult task without outside help.

Brother and sister planned their activities around a tight schedule. The brother lives next door to his mom, and therefore he could quickly come to her aid. As Dementia progresses, the patient cannot be left alone. She cannot cook for herself, bathe or dress herself without help and encouragement.

Both siblings were working, so there was a need for good, dependable help. There are many agencies for the elderly listed in your phonebook, and this is a good place to start. Also, when you network with friends and acquaintances, you will discover loving, competent people who have training and experience caring for Dementia patients. Sometimes, doctors or nurses close to the patient will offer suggestions of caregivers.

Then there are many interviews, backgrounds and references to check. It's quite a job, but in the long run, Dementia patients are calmer and content in their own homes with people they love and/or trust. The siblings have the comfort of knowing their mother/father will be treated with respect and real concern.

Another invaluable resource is Hospice. These wonderful people offer in home care when needed, and free counseling for family members. A nurse will check the patient one to three times a week; a CNA may come to help with baths and dressing. There will be a social worker to help put the program in place and see that all goes well. A chaplain will visit, if the patient and family need some spiritual guidance. Many patients have their own pastors who visit often.

My friend's mother is able to walk, but she has trouble finding her way around a house she has lived in all her life. She is at the stage where she cannot say that she needs to use the potty. And she does not recognize her family. She could fall or wander outside. There are alarms or buzzers available to alert caregivers if a patient gets out of bed or moves from a chair. Doors also have alarms to warn caregivers if a patient tries to go outside unattended.

As I have written, Dementia is an ailment that affects people who have Alzheimer's, Parkinson's and Huntington's disease, as well as Vascular Dementia. All of the above ailments cause the functions of the brain to decline. It's a sad, emotional journey for the patient and her family. A Dementia patient may look the same, but the real person you knew, disappears before your eyes.

How do we cope with the slow death of our loved ones? We try to live life as usual.

We go to work, attend meetings, cook meals, work in the yard and pray a lot. We, as caregivers, must take time for a movie, go out to dinner and get out of town for a day or so. What good are we to our loved ones if we ruin our health trying to do it all? Stop and think. Your sick parent would be the first one to say: "Take it easy, rest," if her mind would allow it.

TIME OUT
FOR CAREGIVERS

If you happen to be the sole caretaker of a loved one, the weight bears heavily on you alone. This is a fact that is evident with each passing day. Everyone will warn you: "You must take care of yourself." You know it's true. But how?

There are resources. Most nursing homes provide a service called Respite Care. The patient may reside in a room, receive his medications by trained personnel, eat his meals, and receive help with all his personal needs. In fact, I know a lady who uses respite every few weeks when she goes to the beach or while she stays at home to rest for a few days. This is a possibility that every caregiver should consider. Not only does your body need to recuperate, your mind needs a rest from responsibility.

When there are others in the family who share the care giving, you are very fortunate. Planning a short vacation is achieved when a brother, sister, child, aunt or uncle gives of their time to care for your loved one for a few days. Each caregiver needs to plan time away from the gloom and sadness that seems to grow when trying to do what is best for your loved one.

Taking care of someone with Dementia is stressful. Caring for a demented patient takes more time than other care giving, and it's definitely a twenty-four hour, seven days a week job. At least 70-80% of care giving is done by family and friends. If funds are available, it is recommended that a professional caregiver be hired to free up the relatives who are responsible for their loved ones. It's easy to burn-out as the same duties are performed over and over. Caregivers feel isolated, many times because of the stigma associated with Dementia. Family and friends do not visit because they don't know what to expect.

It's a helpless feeling to visit a home where a caretaker is struggling with frustration, indecision, feelings of anger and hopelessness. What do you say? How do you encourage caretakers who are so tired, embarrassed by what a loved one does or says, angry and depressed? The person with Dementia is not the person a visitor used to know. The attitude to assume as a visitor is one of positive reinforcement. Smile and speak to the patient and the caregiver. Offer to shake hands with the caregiver while the patient observes. Then, you may offer your hand to the patient. He/she may or may not respond. Accept his behaviors and emotions and don't "back off".

Caretakers need to be able to talk to family and friends about the everyday care of the loved one. One thing is sure, no two days are alike. The caretaker may be angry with the patient because he/she is ill. Maybe she is angry with God. If you are a frequent visitor, listen without judging, show empathy instead of sympathy and let her know that she is always in your thoughts and prayers. Offer some of your time to sit with the patient, or even ask if she would like you to accompany the loved one and her to a doctor's appointment, or to the grocery store.

Shopping while trying to watch a person with Dementia can be a nightmare.

The caregiver may isolate herself and refuse help because she thinks no one really cares about her or her loved one. One solution that may help is to call friends and church members and ask them to send cards of love and cheer. Ask others to show their support by calling or bringing by a favorite dish. Mainly, stay in touch and offer your help and support.

The caregiver cannot escape her responsibilities. She may have a faithful and competent nurse's aide or CNA to shoulder some of the more gruesome tasks of twenty-four care, but still there are many other issues to take valuable time and energy. She will become sleep deprived, have feelings of guilt and impatience and grieve the loss of her personal privacy and space. She may have feelings of conflict about placement issues, disgust with some of the things the patient says or does, or fear for herself. After years of suffering with her loved one, she may wonder if she will ever have a real life again.

People caring for a person who is ill and requires constant care need time alone, time to rest and remember the good years. They need time to attend church services or even a social gathering to see old friends. They need time to pay household bills and shop for food and other necessities. As mentioned earlier, the caregiver must take care of her own health. A caregiver does not have time to be sick, because she is too busy taking care of her loved one. If this describes your situation, you need to take time out to rest and relax as much as possible. The values of respite were stated earlier.

This time of respite cannot be overstated. Your health is a precious commodity. You need good physical and mental health to give the patient the care that he deserves. If the caregiver neglects herself, she may visit the doctor or hospital more than the patient may.

HAVE YOU BEEN DIAGNOSED?

Are you forgetful? Have you had feelings of being lost? Do you have mood changes? Are you able to carry on with your life as usual? Are you frightened? Do you distrust others? Do you feel the need to consult a physician? Have you discussed your feelings with your family? Have they noticed changes that you may have missed?

Dementia is the loss of the ability to think, remember and reason so obvious that it interferes with a person's daily life. Symptoms involve changes in personality, mood and behavior. Dementia occurs when the brain is affected by injury or disease. The most common cause of Dementia is Alzheimer's disease, which accounts for at least half of all cases of Dementia. Most diseases that cause Dementia are not curable; however, about 20% of diseases that cause Dementia are treatable.

Dementia is thought of as a late life disease because it develops mostly in elderly people. About 8% of people over 65 have some form of Dementia. At least half of those over 80 suffer from Dementia. Some types improve with treatment.

The following are treatable:

- Dementia due to drug abuse
- Tumors that can be removed
- Subdural hematoma (usually a head injury)
- Normal-pressure hydrocephalus
- Metabolic disorders (such as the lack of vitamin B)
- Hypothyroidism
- Hypoglycemia.

Dementia that is not treatable:

- Alzheimer's disease
- Multi-infarct Dementia (due to small strokes)
- Dementia of Parkinson's disease
- AIDS Dementia.

Some doctors will prescribe medicine to help the patient cope, but there are no lasting benefits.

The first sign of early of Dementia is usually memory loss. The difference between Dementia and normal forgetfulness is that the memory loss is constant. Friends begin to notice changes in behavior on a social level.

THE DEEP WELL OF FORGETFULNESS

My friend, Martha, once told me how sad she is to realize that her mother is not able to carry on a meaningful conversation. Like many of us, Martha has been accustomed to sharing her joys and sorrows with a mother who enjoyed being kept up to date with her family. Her mom was someone she could go to for advice or a hug when she needed it. Martha was accustomed to confiding in her mother, and she valued her opinion. She grew up thinking that her mom would always have a solution or a least suggestions on solving life's problems. However, Martha expressed her frustration because her mother looks the same but she is a totally different person.

This "person" cannot understand Martha or carry on a conversation with her. Even worse, her mother does not seem to know exactly who Martha is. As her mom's Dementia grew worse, Martha began to miss the daily telephone conversations they had shared. Her mother has no idea what a phone is or how to use it. As she wanders around the house, she picks up objects, looks at them and places them back. Martha thinks that her mom knows that many things look familiar, but her mind cannot provide an answer.

Martha's mom has been evaluated by doctors who say that she has cognitive problems. Cognitive means to know. Cognitive skills are important in everyday life because they cause the brain to perceive, to reason, to remember, to come to conclusions, to understand and to have insight. Without these skills, it is impossible to live a normal life. It's these very cognitive skills that make us who we are to others. The body can be the same, but vital parts of the mind are buried in darkness.

It must be so frightening to not know where you are, you may look all around, trying to recognize something or someone. What a desperate feeling! Your heart pounds. You are scared. When you have Dementia, you are lost forever.

Patients who suffer from Dementia must be in a calm and loving environment, which offers lots of support for the patient and his caregivers. Martha and her father began seeking a facility that could care for her mother as her condition worsened. They visited a nursing home with a Memory Care Unit. The patients seemed well supervised, and the atmosphere was calm and pleasant. They spoke with the staff and director. Over the next several months, Martha and/or her father became very familiar with the Memory Care Unit and compared it with others nearby. Meanwhile, the mother's personality changed from low-key to energy-charged. It was becoming very difficult for two caregivers to keep up with her and care for all her daily needs.

When the time came for the move to the facility, Martha and her father were ready. They spent many hours making their loved one's room so very much like home. Much of her furniture from home was placed in the room along with pictures on the walls. Many family pictures were placed in frames on shelves, and her closet was filled with her own clothing. On moving day, Martha placed her mom in her favorite recliner, which faced her own television set. She seemed to feel at home. Nurses coming in and out of her room seemed like the routine at home.

Martha and her father breathed a sigh of relief knowing that their loved one would get her medicine on time and be well cared for by people who were trained to work with Dementia patients. They will know what to do when the mother becomes angry or combative. The staff will see that the patient gets exercise, the correct food and plenty of activities to keep her busy. Martha and her father made a commitment to visit their loved one every day, each at different times. By doing this, they will know how their patient is progressing, and hopefully surprise her with a familiar face. It's not an easy task to place a family member in a facility. Careful investigation and thought must play a part in the decision. The goal is to get the best care possible, and keep the patient as content as possible. A caring, loving family will go the extra mile to make the transition work.

While visiting Care Facilities in an official and personal capacity, I have sadly noticed that our elderly population is being placed in Care Facility Homes and forgotten. The patients and nurses will agree that many of the sick and elderly have no visitors for weeks, months, or never. It is a disgrace that we dishonor our elders so badly. The other side of the coin is when the sick and elderly remain at home only to be abused by their own families. As the population ages, I am afraid that the problem will only worsen.

DEPENDING ON SITTERS TO CARE FOR YOUR PARENT

The truth of the matter is that you can't totally depend on sitters to care for your loved one. You will find that people who are nursing assistants, those who have had some experience caring for the elderly, and those who will merely watch your parent are hard to find. Each person has his own set of family obligations, sicknesses and unique personalities, which sometimes can jumble up a well-planned schedule of care for your loved-one. One schedule of caring qualified caregivers may be valid for only two weeks. Then, you begin consulting your remaining list of possibilities.

When you begin to realize that that your parent needs help at home, the search begins. First, inquire at your local Hospice Home. Many times, they have a list of qualified people who are looking for a part-time job. They may suggest someone who will live-in on a twenty-four hour bases. Look in the phone book for Elder Care and Adult Care Services. Call anyone you may know who has an elderly parent and uses the services of paid caretakers. Visit local nursing homes, and talk to those in charge. They usually know of some CNA (certified nursing assistant) who would be interested in working an extra eight to ten hours a week. The hospitals usually have a list of caretakers. The possibilities are endless. So network, network, and then network some more.

When you have a list of names and numbers, the tough work begins. Any prospect will need to meet with you and your parent. She should spend at least two hours visiting with your loved one. Ask for references, and check them out. For safety sake, a criminal background check is in order.

At the time of her visit with your parent, explain just what is expected of her as a caretaker. Tell her about your parent's personality, the medicines she takes, her daily habits, and explain any food likes and dislikes. Talk about the hours the caretaker will be needed and try to come together on an hourly wage or lump sum payment per day. Even after you are satisfied, and she begins work, there should be a trial period of one to two weeks. This is necessary because your parent may decide she does not like the caretaker; the caretaker may display some characteristics that are not pleasant, or the caretaker may decide she does not like the position.

It's always helpful to make up menus that your parent will eat, and keep all these items in stock at all times. Let the caretaker know how your parent likes his coffee, how he likes his food cooked and what consistency the food should be. The doctors will determine if there is a swallowing problem, and if there is, he will suggest the correct liquidity for the food. Pharmacies and home health stores sell a gel-like substance that makes eating safer for the sick and elderly.

List names and phone numbers of people to call if the caretaker has a simple question or if there is an emergency. If there is a problem, always stress that the caretakers call 911 first, and then call a family member or friend who lives close by. Keeping satisfactory help is a continuous process of networking, interviewing, checking references and being sure to hire a caretaker who will interact well with the patient.

If your loved one does not care for the caretaker, she will let you know with various signs or changes in her behavior. She may be combative, use foul language or withdraw in silence. When you notice negative changes in your loved one, you must replace the caretaker.

Part III

Day to Day Care

DEMENTIA CANNOT BE DELAYED OR CURED

When a patient is diagnosed with any form of Dementia, many doctors will prescribe medications to temporarily improve some memory processes. You may discover that your patient cannot tolerate some of the medicines because of the side effects. However, if the primary care doctor prescribes a medicine that may keep your loved one's mind more lucid, try it. As I've said before, NEVER GIVE UP. The new medicine may help for a while, and make life easier for the patient and caregivers. Just remember, there is not yet any medicine that can cure Dementia or slow it's progress. The best medicine caretakers and family members can give is love and patience.

Prescribed medicines that seem most valuable are those that calm anxieties, and help with sleep. Anti-depressants may be used for anti-social behavior problems. As the disease progresses there are secondary illnesses to be aware of.

When someone is ill with Dementia or any other terminal disease, his status of health will change without warning. Other than the different phases of any chronic disease, there are complications of infections and dehydration. Older adults tend to easily become dehydrated because they forget to drink enough water. Evidence shows that a person who has a mind-altering disease must be offered water and other liquids several times a day. Caretakers should observe while a patient consumes the liquids and record the amount. Dehydration in someone who is very sick and/or elderly is dangerous. There may be several times that your loved one will be hospitalized because of dehydration. A nurse at a care facility once told me that more residents go to the hospital because of dehydration than any other single ailment.

One of the most common infections that plague patients is urinary tract infections or UTI's.

Your loved one may not complain of aches and pains, so the caretakers (or you) must watch for signs of agitation and periods of sleepiness. He/she may rub her lower stomach, the urine may have a strong odor and/or the urine may be dark, not pale yellow. In view of these events, the patient must see his/her primary care doctor.

When the doctor prescribes an antibiotic because of a UTI or any other infection, a patient may develop a yeast infection at any warm and moist part of his/her body. You may notice redness and a rash in the private areas that will get worse unless treated properly. A call to the doctor or triage nurse will get the care the patient needs.

All caretakers need to watch for pressure sores, also called skin breakdown and bedsores. This ailment is a devastating development for one who is struggling with a terminal disease. Older patients who are not mobile will often have this problem. Patients sit most of the day in wheelchairs; some cannot even change their position as people normally do. Other patients lie in bed and must be turned at least every two hours to prevent or relieve pressure sores. Tender skin will wrinkle, or scrape lightly against a sheet or pad, which could cause skin breakdown. Such a condition must be taken care of immediately. In home care facilities, there are special nurses who deal with this problem on a daily basis. If your loved one is in Hospice, their nurse will care for bedsores. However, if your parent is at home, you must take him/her to the primary care doctor for treatment.

Bedsores can be prevented whether the patient is at home or in a facility. During daily baths, the patients' skin must be inspected carefully for red spots, scrapes, deep wrinkles (caused by sheets or pads that are not smooth), and small breaks. The patient must be thoroughly dried after a bath and/or after a change of underwear. A special cream, sometimes called *fanny cream,* must be applied at least twice a day. If the breakdown gets worse, a doctor must be consulted immediately. Infection can enter any open wound on a patient's body. Patients with bedsores are usually in a lot of pain, but they cannot express it.

Care must be taken when feeding someone with Dementia. As the disease progresses, patients find it difficult to swallow. Even a simple sip of water will sometimes stay in the mouth until it dribbles out or trickles down the throat and causes the patient to strangle. If water or food enters the lung area it can cause infection such as pneumonia. Caregivers should take particular precautions to encourage their patients to swallow, or at least offer a container so the patients can spit out the substance. Many Dementia patients have something added to their food and drink to prevent choking. Many stores make this "thickening" available without a prescription.

As the disease progresses, even daily medicines will be difficult to swallow. Crushing pills and giving them in yogurt, applesauce or pudding helps for a while. Some medicines come in liquid form, which may help. But finally, all medicines will be eliminated because of the danger of not swallowing properly, and/or the patient will refuse to open his/her mouth.

THE DOCTOR AND PHARMACIST ARE FRIENDS YOU NEED

Always have heart-to-heart discussions with all the doctors who are treating your parent. I know this request is one that will try your patience, as well as the doctors'. When you have seen doctors hurry from one patient to the next, it seems impossible to ask questions that are so necessary for your parents care. But don't let that stop you. I have chased doctors down the hall while calling their names. I've never had one to ignore me. I am persistent because I want the best care for my parent, and so do you.

Being persistent also means many medical appointments, making numerous phone calls and requesting material that the doctors may have on hand that pertain to your parent's illness. Ask for any information that may help your parent cope with Dementia and other diseases that affect the elderly. Don't worry about making the doctor angry; he'll get over it. When you show your true concern by asking questions, medical professionals will know that you are sincere. This is not the last time I will say this: ALWAYS SHOW YOUR LOVE AND CONCERN FOR YOUR PARENT, AND NEVER GIVE UP. Don't hesitate to ask for a second opinion. Most physicians expect families to cover all bases.

As I emphasized earlier, keep a log and use it. Use it to review your notes from previous visits, to record medicine changes and to add any new directions from the doctor. Share this information with your parent's other caretakers. If later, you have questions, call the physician's office and ask for help. A triage nurse will be glad to speak with you. Remember, your goal is to learn everything possible to make life easier for your parent.

Another suggestion is to make friends with your pharmacist. Talk with him when you pick up medications; ask about side effects, the best time of day to give the medicine, and what to do if too much is taken by mistake. Many times doctors do not go into detail about such things, and you will discover that your pharmacist is a wealth of information. You may ask if a certain medicine has a generic equivalent, to save money on the many medicines an older person needs. I have found that the smaller pharmacies are more helpful, tend to give better service, and *some still deliver to your home.* Also, if you ask, the smaller pharmacies will usually meet the lower prices of generic drugs sold in the larger stores. Don't hesitate. Always ask! THERE IS NO STUPID QUESTION.

With the help of a friendly pharmacist, select a large pillbox that has clear markings as of time and day. Better still, get a box with no markings, and make your own as needed. This enables the caretaker to give the correct dosage at the correct time, without fail. A seven-day box, divided into four compartments for each day works very well, but your needs may be different. Have that friendly pharmacist or his/her assistant help you select. PRN (as needed) medicine needs to be kept together in a safe place so as not to be confused with daily meds. The caregiver who goes to the doctor with the patient should be the one to fill the pillbox. All other caretakers should be advised about the medicines, where they are kept and how to administer them.

CARING FOR YOUR PARENT AT HOME

As mentioned earlier, many Dementia patients are able to live at home for many years. Careful planning and organization is necessary to meet the needs of the patient and insure a safe and tranquil atmosphere. Plans should be made considering the parent's usual lifestyle. Times for eating, hobbies (former interest), familiar television programs, reading the newspaper, napping and bedtime should follow the same pattern as set by the parent before her illness. The calmer the surroundings, the more peaceful and cooperative the patient will be. He/she must feel secure, safe and loved.

If the patient is mobile and walks around a lot, there must be locks on the doors with keys he cannot use. An all power hospital bed with side rails should be obtained. Medicare will pay for a bed and other needed equipment if you ask the doctor to prescribe it. An alarm system can be installed on the doors, on the bed and on the wheelchair to signal that the patient is moving. These devices are easily found at nearby home health stores, or through your pharmacy. You can do a Web search for home health on your computer and get whatever you need.

If your parent tends to wander it will usually be when he/she is not busy. Try to have an activity (drawing, coloring, looking at a magazine together or a favorite television program) or offer a snack your parent/patient particularly likes. As you try to engage your parent in conversation, or an activity, please speak calmly and clearly. Repeat yourself if necessary, but not in an impatient voice. Stand beside the person, and explain what you want him/her to do.

Being calm and not hasty in movement works very well when bathing, helping with the toilet and dressing your loved one. ALWAYS explain in a clear calm voice what you are going to help her do. If you don't, she may resist, bite or hit you. Being gentle and loving will usually discourage any negative behavior.

Probably the most difficult part of keeping Mom at home will be finding a qualified, trust-worthy person to help care for her. As you interview people, explain her/his illness. Choose someone who has worked with Dementia or Alzheimer's patients. Ask for references, and call each one. As you discuss your parent's needs, be sure the aid understands all that is involved in the care of him.

When you hire an aid (CNA), have a family member stay with her for a few days, so that she will learn your routine, your parent's ways, medicines to give and when, foods she likes, and explain the calm atmosphere that keeps your parent happy and manageable. He/she must be able to prepare meals, bathe and dress your parent. Salary and schedules must be agreed upon if all goes well. You may interview eight or ten people before you find one that fits. One of the most important traits an aid must have is DEPENDABILITY.

FRANK LOST HIMSELF

Frank was a man who was well thought of in his community, his church and in the workplace. His job required him to travel, but he was always glad to return home to his wife and sons. The job was one that consisted of meetings and classes designed to learn more about the product. He eventually rose to the position of manager. He was a very personable man, and got along well with others. As Frank reached middle-age he spoke to his wife about slowing down the pace of his job. He had noticed that his coworkers were not as friendly as they had been. Maybe it was because their names occasionally escaped his usually brilliant mind. He didn't feel like a leader anymore. Simple problems were vague and impossible to solve.

Elizabeth, Frank's wife, was puzzled by Frank's lack of interest when planning his next trip. He contacted the usual co-workers to discuss dates and times; however, he sat at his desk unsure of what he would do next. Frank knew where he was going, but he was undecided about what transportation he would use. He sat for long periods with his head in his hands, trying to make sense of what he was supposed to do.

Elizabeth was in their bedroom packing clothes for a five-day trip as she had done for many years. This trip just did not feel right. Should she ask Frank not to go? A feeling of gloom and knowing flooded her mind and heart. The husband she had depended on was now depending on her. Close friends had hinted that Frank was not the man they had known. If Elizabeth were being truthful with herself, she would agree.

She called a friend who was a nurse and described her fears. She urged Elizabeth to get Frank to a doctor right away. Elizabeth loved her husband, and she was afraid that he was changing forever. Life had been so calm and pleasant as the couple planned trips they wanted to take during retirement. Life changes overnight and we are never ready.

She found Frank as she had left him, sitting at his desk with a far off look on his face. She asked him to cancel his trip, and to her relief, he agreed. Tomorrow she would call the doctor and brace for the truth. The journey lay ahead.

The doctor gave Frank a physical and many tests to check his memory and cognitive ability. Word and number games were used to check his short-term memory. The time of day, the day of the week, the month of the year, his birthday, the president's name, the current year and his age were some questions asked of Frank. There were written tests, and other verbal exercises. Frank was frustrated and looked repeatedly to Elizabeth for help. He was later referred to a geriatric specialist who diagnosed him with Alzheimer's disease.

Elizabeth was devastated. She called their sons and other family members. They offered words of encouragement and support. Elizabeth tried to keep the same routine. She continued choir practice while one of the boys stayed with their father. She went to the hairdresser, and did her shopping. Frank asked for her while she was gone, but she needed the time to think and gather the strength that she needed to face the next day. She was brave, but she also knew that every day was uncertain and no two days are alike. She learned not to expect any improvement, or bolt of lightning changes. She was grateful when Frank remembered her name, when he smiled at her, and when he ate a good meal.

"One day at a time" was her motto.

Frank and Elizabeth continued to attend church, go to social gatherings and enjoy quiet times together. As the months passed, Elizabeth began to grow weary of bathing, dressing and all the other personal things she was doing for Frank. He was a large man who could not help himself, and Elizabeth needed all the help she could get. A friend recommended a caregiver who turned out to be a lifesaver. As Frank became weaker and less cooperative, a male nurse was hired to work with him.

Frank's family was so sad to see how this strong, outgoing man was reduced to a shell of the person he was. His eyes held no expression. His face was pale and drawn. He did not acknowledge people who came to see him. His brain could not make any sense of his surroundings or the words that people were throwing at him. He could not find his way. Frank had lost himself.

WHEN THE SYSTEM BREAKS DOWN

Speaking from experience, there will be a day when the well thought out schedule will be useless. Just today, a lady who we found through Hospice decided not to show up for work. My brother and I had interviewed her for three hours while she was at Mom's house. She met Mom, we talked about Mom's daily routine, we discussed medicines, she practiced moving Mom from one chair to another, she gave us references and a salary was agreed upon. I checked her references, and no one said anything negative. I called her a few days later and asked her to work Wednesday and Thursday of the next week. She agreed, but she called me on Monday of that week to ask questions about her salary. I repeated what we had decided on the day of her interview. She felt that it was not enough money, so I offered her more. She wanted to discuss it with her husband, and she waited until Tuesday night to call me telling me she could not work with us.

I am sitting now with mother waiting for one of our good helpers to arrive. This lady is a CNA who also works in a nursing home. She and mother get along very well, and this is not the first time that she has come to our rescue. This lady always goes the extra mile by doing extra things for mom. She reads to mother and tries to carry on a conversation with her. Most importantly, we trust her with mother.

Since no one is perfect, I'm not surprised when our CNA comes in late. Sometimes she may be as late as two hours. We continue to call her because it's difficult to get someone on short notice, and she is good at what she does. The ideal situation is one where the same person stays 24/7. Almost as good, is to have two caretakers who stay 12 hours each.

BRENDA'S LAST DAYS

The loving care given to Brenda during her decline was ending. Brenda knew when it all started. She drove into a shopping center with which she was familiar. Yet, nothing looked the same. Brenda was afraid. Where was she and how would she get home?

Then one day she could not remember how to stop the car she was driving. Of course, there was a collision. She was trying to cope with a husband who's health was declining. There was stress and sadness in her everyday life. Brenda seemed to withdraw and was unusually quiet. As the months passed, she forgot things from the recent past and even things from her youth. Brenda spent most days searching for something.

She emptied every drawer in her house, still looking. Sometimes she would say what she was trying to find; other times she did not know. She usually folded the clothes nicely and returned them to the drawers. There were times when she put things in the dryer or freezer for no reason. She had lots of anxiety, and at times, she would strike out at a caregiver while saying ugly words. Her caregiver was not shocked or surprised.

All these actions are characteristic of a Dementia patient. She endured several stitches and two broken bones from frequent falls. One head injury caused her Dementia to worsen. When she was released from the hospital following her last injury, Brenda's family took her back home.

She seemed content to sit in her special recliner, look at the paper, watch television or nap. As months passed, Brenda forgot many things. She forgot how to walk and the names of family and friends. But she usually had a smile for her visitors.

It was a challenge to find reliable help, rearrange the house, and get all the things needed to care for someone who could not walk without help. Family members changed their schedules to be with Brenda as much as possible. Several CNA's were interviewed and before long, Brenda had a caregiver who also became her friend. The weeks became months, and the months became years. Brenda was content being home where her friends and family could easily visit. She talked very little.

As time passed, there were many trips to the doctor and/or the hospital. There were blood clots and numerous infections. At times, the doctors were amazed when Brenda was able to bounce back. But each illness took its toll on her general health, and her Dementia steadily worsened. Her Primary Care Physician was encouraging, and commented to her family about the unselfish love and care they gave their mother.

After Brenda's health began to decline more rapidly, her PCP called in Hospice. Her family was grateful for the extra help, even though they knew that Hospice was usually called in to make dying patients comfortable.

The Hospice nurses, nursing assistants, the Chaplin and the social workers were wonderful, supportive people. They were sure that Brenda had the medicine and other supplies she needed. They counseled Brenda's family about "the end of life experience." Even though the family did not want to let Brenda go, they knew that the time was near.

During the last three weeks of her life, Brenda never left her bed. She had been eating very well until she forgot how to swallow. She would spit out her medicine and hold food in her mouth. They tried thickened liquids, but nothing seemed to work. Finally, Brenda refused to open her mouth. She stopped talking and just slept. Brenda was without food or drink for fourteen days before she passed away.

At the beginning of Brenda's decline, she would smile at her family. She did not move unless a caretaker would actually turn her over to make her more comfortable. Pillows were put to her back and between her legs. Hospice nurses, caretakers and family members were very mindful of the dangers of little wrinkles in such thin skin. Bedsores (ulcers) develop easily when a patient lies or sits in the same position for as little as thirty minutes. They, most commonly, appear on the back, buttocks, legs and feet and they are very painful. They must be treated by keeping the area clean, using special medication and changing dressing frequently.

During her last few days, Brenda mouthed "thank you" to her family and caretakers. When she heard her children's voices, she opened her eyes and held up her arms to hug them. She kissed them with dry lips that had not tasted water in days. It was such a precious time for her family, even though they knew that Brenda was saying "good-bye."

While her favorite hymns played softly, she was getting ready. She was comfortable, warm, and out of pain. Her breathing pattern changed, from regular to slower and less regular. Her face was serene. She took a long breath, and slipped away as her children held her hands and bade her "good-bye."

HELP WHEN YOU NEED IT

Below you will find helpful organizations and internet links as you face the challenge of dealing with someone with Dementia.

Depression in the elderly:
www.nami.org/helpline/elddepres.htm

Seniors Internet Resource Center:
www.ageofreason.com

Dealing with Dementia:
www.nepamd.com/Dementia.htm

Vascular Dementia (or multi-infarct Dementia):
http://helpguide.org/elder/vascular

Boomer Books contain practical knowledge and solutions for dealing with family, retirement, and aging: http://boomer-books.com/Dementia/

Information on transient ischemic attack (TIA) sometimes called a mini-stroke. A TIA is often a warning sign of a stroke and must not be ignored:
http://www.closurei.com/patient/stroketia/tia.html

If you are concerned your loved one may be in the early stages of Alzheimer's disease, learn more about the symptoms:
http://www.everydayhealth.com/health-report

A symptom screener can help you identify whether a problem may exist, however, only a doctor can diagnose Alzheimer's or any other type of Dementia:
http://.alzheimersrxtreatment.com

Free information and helpful suggestions—The Alzheimer's Association
http://www.alz.org

Alzheimer's Association help line-(703)359-4440
www.mayoclinic.com/health/alzheimers-disease

Information about the problems that accompany our aging population: National Institute on Aging (1-301-496-1752) www.nia.nih.gov

Help caring for patients with Dementia: National Hospice and Palliative Care Organization (1-703-837-1500), www.nhpco.org

Help for veterans and their spouses: Veterans Administration www.va.gov. This site can put you in touch with your local VA office, so that you can make an appointment to answer questions about your specific financial needs. Your local Congressman will be glad to help expedite the process.

For Assisted Living:
www.assisted-living-directory.com

GLOSSARY OF WORDS PRETAINING TO ELDERLY PATIENT

Activities of Daily Living (ADL)-Everyday personal tasks that are required for people to live on their own such as: the ability to feed oneself, go to the toilet, take a bath or get out of bed.

Acute—A sudden and severe condition.

Adult day services—A facility where older adults who need supervision may interact with other adults for a few hours a day.

Advance directives (living will)—Informs the family of your wishes in a medical emergency.

Age Associated Memory Impairment—Mild memory loss that increases with age. Mild memory loss is normal and should not be confused with forms of dementia.

Amyloidal plaque-Buildup of amyloidal protein in someone with Alzheimer's.

Anti-anxiety drug—A drug given to ease anxiety of a patient.

Anti-psychotic drug—Used to manage behavior problems for patients with serious mental disorders.

Age—associated Memory Impairment—Mild memory loss that increases with age and should not be confused with forms of dementia.

Alzheimer's Disease—Symptoms include: short term memory loss, difficulty solving problems, inability to perform familiar tasks, time related confusion, visions problems and word confusion.

Ambulate—To walk

Antibiotic—Drug used to treat infections.

Assisted Living—Is a senior living option that combines housing, support services and health care as needed.

Asphyxia—Occurs when one stops breathing and the heart stops beating.

Assessment—Determination of a patient's care needs based on a formal evaluation.

Atrophy—Cell loss in the body because of age or lack of use.

Bed Sores/Pressure Ulcers—When patients stay in bed in one position for long periods of time their skin becomes raw and red. Little abrasions appear, and they develop into major sores if not treated. That is why bed—ridden people must be turned at least every two hours.

Bereavement Counseling—Psychotherapy or supportive counseling that is designed to help people come to terms with the loss of significant others in their lives.

CNA—Certified Nurse Assistants

Case Management—The practice of having a single expert, often a social worker, psychologist, counselor, or a nurse, who works with the client, family and other professionals involved with a case to plan and coordinate some or all of the health and social services needed by the client.

DSS—Department of Social Services

DHHS—US Department of Health and Human Services

Dementia—Collection of symptoms including memory loss, personality change, and impaired intellectual functions resulting from disease or trauma to the brain. These changes are not part of normal aging and are severe enough to impact daily living, independence, and relationships.

Durable Power of Attorney—A legal document giving another person authority to make financial and legal decisions if the principal becomes physically or mentally incompetent.

Elder Abuse—Any physical abuse, sexual abuse, abandonment, isolation, neglect, financial abuse of an older or dependent person.

EMT—Emergency Medical Technician

Geriatrics—The branch of medicine that focuses on providing health care for the elderly and the treatment of diseases associated with the aging process

Geriatrician—The physician who specializes in the practice of geriatrics.

Gerontology—Scientific study of the process and problems of aging.

Gerontologist—A specialist in gerontology.

GI tube—a tube inserted surgically through an opening in the stomach. GI tubes offer another means of nutritional sustenance for those individuals unable to take these substances by mouth.

Guardianship—An extreme measure that severely restricts the legal rights of an elder based on a court's finding of legal incompetence. Another individual is assigned the responsibility of handling the elder person's legal affairs.

Health Care Directive—A written legal document which allows a person to appoint another person (agent) to make health care decisions should he or she is unable to make or communicate decisions.

Health Care Power of Attorney—The appointment of a health care agent to make decisions when the person becomes unable to make or communicate.

Home Health Aide—Provides personal care and help with monitoring medications, exercises and other assistance for a disabled elderly person.

Hospice—Hospice/Palliative care is provided to enhance the life of the dying person. Typically offered in the last 6 months of life, emphasizes comfort measures and counseling to provide social, spiritual and physical support to the dying patient and his or her family.

Hospice Care—the provision of short-term inpatient services for pain control and management of symptoms related to terminal illness.

Lifeline—A telephone alert system that enables elderly persons who live alone to receive help in a medical emergency.

Living Will—A general written statement specifying or limiting medical treatment. It is an official legal document, but different states have different requirements about witnesses and other rules under which a living will is acceptable.

Physical Therapist (PT)—A person professionally trained in the practice of physical therapy.

Respite Services—Support for a family member or other caregiver who is assisting someone with a serious medical condition or dementia.

Respite is designed to help the family members get a break from their caregiver responsibilities. Respite care may entail the patient entering a facility for a short stay or it may be services provided by an in home attendant or day care program.

Senior Centers—These programs are sometimes called Multi-purpose Senior Centers. They provide older adults who are not home bound the opportunity for social interaction in a centralized location via a variety of activities and programs.

Skilled Nursing Facility (SNF)—A state licensed medical facility that provides services for rehabilitation or for long-term care. Often they are called nursing homes or convalescent hospitals.

Speech Therapist—A specially trained professional person who specializes in helping a person regain speech after suffering from stroke or other debilitating condition. A speech therapist also has training to provide care for a patient who has difficulty in swallowing.

Supplemental Security Income (SSI)—A monthly cash grant provided to eligible individuals who have particularly low income and assets.

Supportive Services—A range of supports including home attendant care, home health care, adult day care, case management, counseling, legal assistance, meal programs, transportation, and other designed to help an older or disabled adult maintain their highest level of functioning and remain safely in the home.

TIA—Mini strokes in the brain that cause Vascular Dementia.

Vascular Dementia—Blood vessels in the brain that have clots that break loose and cause TIA'S.